FINAL REPORT OF THE NATIONAL ACADEMIES' HUMAN EMBRYONIC STEM CELL RESEARCH ADVISORY COMMITTEE AND 2010 AMENDMENTS TO THE NATIONAL ACADEMIES' GUIDELINES FOR HUMAN EMBRYONIC STEM CELL RESEARCH

Human Embryonic Stem Cell Research Advisory Committee

Board on Life Sciences
Division on Earth and Life Studies

Board on Health Sciences Policy
Institute of Medicine

NATIONAL RESEARCH COUNCIL *AND*
INSTITUTE OF MEDICINE
OF THE NATIONAL ACADEMIES

THE NATIONAL ACADEMIES PRESS
Washington, D.C.
www.nap.edu

THE NATIONAL ACADEMIES PRESS 500 Fifth Street, NW Washington, DC 20001

NOTICE: The project that is the subject of this report was approved by the Governing Board of the National Research Council, whose members are drawn from the councils of the National Academy of Sciences, the National Academy of Engineering, and the Institute of Medicine. The members of the committee responsible for the report were chosen for their special competences and with regard for appropriate balance.

This study was supported by The Ellison Medical Foundation. Any opinions, findings, conclusions, or recommendations expressed in this publication are those of the authors and do not necessarily reflect the views of the organizations or agencies that provided support for the project.

International Standard Book Number-13: 978-0-309-15600-4
International Standard Book Number-10: 0-309-15600-9

Additional copies of this report are available from the National Academies Press, 500 Fifth Street, NW, Lockbox 285, Washington, DC 20055; (800) 624-6242 or (202) 334-3313 (in the Washington metropolitan area); Internet, http://www.nap.edu.

Suggested citation: National Research Council and Institute of Medicine. 2010. *Final Report of the National Academies' Human Embryonic Stem Cell Research Advisory Committee and 2010 Amendments to the National Academies' Guidelines for Human Embryonic Stem Cell Research*. Washington, DC: The National Academies Press.

Cover: A cluster of motor neurons and neural fibers derived from human embryonic stem cells in the lab of University of Wisconsin-Madison stem cell researcher and neurodevelopmental biologist Su-Chan Zhang. These motor neurons were developed from one of James Thomson's original human embryonic stem cell lines. Copyright for the photograph is held by the University of Wisconsin's Board of Regents.

Additional copies of this report are available from the National Academies Press, 500 Fifth Street, NW, Lockbox 285, Washington, DC 20055; (800) 624-6242 or (202) 334-3313 (in the Washington metropolitan area); Internet, http://www.nap.edu.

Printed in the United States of America

THE NATIONAL ACADEMIES

Advisers to the Nation on Science, Engineering, and Medicine

The **National Academy of Sciences** is a private, nonprofit, self-perpetuating society of distinguished scholars engaged in scientific and engineering research, dedicated to the furtherance of science and technology and to their use for the general welfare. Upon the authority of the charter granted to it by the Congress in 1863, the Academy has a mandate that requires it to advise the federal government on scientific and technical matters. Dr. Ralph J. Cicerone is president of the National Academy of Sciences.

The **National Academy of Engineering** was established in 1964, under the charter of the National Academy of Sciences, as a parallel organization of outstanding engineers. It is autonomous in its administration and in the selection of its members, sharing with the National Academy of Sciences the responsibility for advising the federal government. The National Academy of Engineering also sponsors engineering programs aimed at meeting national needs, encourages education and research, and recognizes the superior achievements of engineers. Dr. Charles Vest is president of the National Academy of Engineering.

The **Institute of Medicine** was established in 1970 by the National Academy of Sciences to secure the services of eminent members of appropriate professions in the examination of policy matters pertaining to the health of the public. The Institute acts under the responsibility given to the National Academy of Sciences by its congressional charter to be an adviser to the federal government and, upon its own initiative, to identify issues of medical care, research, and education. Dr. Harvey V. Fineberg is president of the Institute of Medicine.

The **National Research Council** was organized by the National Academy of Sciences in 1916 to associate the broad community of science and technology with the Academy's purposes of furthering knowledge and advising the federal government. Functioning in accordance with general policies determined by the Academy, the Council has become the principal operating agency of both the National Academy of Sciences and the National Academy of Engineering in providing services to the government, the public, and the scientific and engineering communities. The Council is administered jointly by both Academies and the Institute of Medicine. Dr. Ralph J. Cicerone and Dr. Charles Vest are chair and vice chair, respectively, of the National Research Council.

www.national-academies.org

HUMAN EMBRYONIC STEM CELL RESEARCH ADVISORY COMMITTEE

R. ALTA CHARO (*Co-chair*), University of Wisconsin, Madison, WI[1]
RICHARD O. HYNES (*Co-chair*), Howard Hughes Medical Institute and Massachusetts Institute of Technology, Cambridge, MA
ELI Y. ADASHI, Brown University, Providence, RI
BRIGID L.M. HOGAN, Duke University Medical Center, Durham, NC
MARCIA IMBRESCIA, Peartree Design, Lynnfield, MA
TERRY MAGNUSON, University of North Carolina, Chapel Hill, NC
LINDA B. MILLER, Volunteer Trustees Foundation, Washington, DC
JONATHAN D. MORENO, University of Pennsylvania, Philadelphia, PA
PILAR N. OSSORIO, University of Wisconsin, Madison, WI
E. ALBERT REECE, University of Maryland, Baltimore, MD
JOSHUA R. SANES, Harvard University, Cambridge, MA
HAROLD T. SHAPIRO, Princeton University, Princeton, NJ
JOHN E. WAGNER, Jr., University of Minnesota, Minneapolis, MN

Staff

ADAM P. FAGEN, Senior Program Officer, Board on Life Sciences
BRUCE M. ALTEVOGT, Senior Program Officer, Board on Health Sciences Policy
FRANCES E. SHARPLES, Director, Board on Life Sciences
ANDREW M. POPE, Director, Board on Health Sciences Policy
AMANDA P. CLINE, Senior Program Assistant, Board on Life Sciences

[1] Professor Charo was appointed as a senior policy advisor in the Office of the Commissioner of the U.S. Food and Drug Administration (FDA) on August 31, 2009. None of her assigned tasks at FDA are related to the topics discussed in this report.

BOARD ON LIFE SCIENCES

KEITH YAMAMOTO (*Chair*), University of California, San Francisco, CA
ANN M. ARVIN, Stanford University, Stanford, CA
BONNIE L. BASSLER, Howard Hughes Medical Institute and Princeton University, Princeton, NJ
VICKI L. CHANDLER, Gordon and Betty Moore Foundation, Palo Alto, CA
SEAN EDDY, Janelia Farm Research Campus, Howard Hughes Medical Institute, Ashburn, VA
MARK D. FITZSIMMONS, John D. and Catherine T. MacArthur Foundation, Chicago, IL
DAVID R. FRANZ, Midwest Research Institute, Frederick, MD
LOUIS J. GROSS, University of Tennessee, Knoxville, TN
JO HANDELSMAN, Yale University, New Haven, CT
CATO T. LAURENCIN, University of Connecticut Health Center, Farmington, CT
JONATHAN D. MORENO, University of Pennsylvania, Philadelphia, PA
ROBERT M. NEREM, Georgia Institute of Technology, Atlanta, GA
CAMILLE PARMESAN, University of Texas, Austin, TX
MURIEL E. POSTON, Skidmore College, Saratoga Springs, NY
ALISON G. POWER, Cornell University, Ithaca, NY
BRUCE W. STILLMAN, Cold Spring Harbor Laboratory, Cold Spring Harbor, NY
CYNTHIA WOLBERGER, Howard Hughes Medical Institute and Johns Hopkins University School of Medicine, Baltimore, MD
MARY WOOLLEY, Research!America, Alexandria, VA

Staff

FRANCES E. SHARPLES, Director
JO L. HUSBANDS, Scholar/Senior Project Director
KATHERINE BOWMAN, Senior Program Officer
ADAM P. FAGEN, Senior Program Officer
MARILEE K. SHELTON-DAVENPORT, Senior Program Officer
INDIA HOOK-BARNARD, Program Officer
ANNA FARRAR, Financial Associate
CARL-GUSTAV ANDERSON, Senior Program Assistant
AMANDA P. CLINE, Senior Program Assistant
AMANDA MAZZAWI, Program Assistant

Acknowledgments

The Committee acknowledges the input received from members of the stem cell research and oversight communities and the speakers and participants in its meetings.

This report has been reviewed in draft form by individuals chosen for their diverse perspectives and technical expertise, in accordance with procedures approved by the National Research Council's Report Review Committee. The purpose of this independent review is to provide candid and critical comments that will assist the institution in making its published report as sound as possible and to ensure that the report meets institutional standards for objectivity, evidence, and responsiveness to the study charge. The review comments and draft manuscript remain confidential to protect the integrity of the deliberative process. We wish to thank the following individuals for their review of this report:

George Q. Daley, Howard Hughes Medical Institute, Children's Hospital Boston, and Harvard Medical School
Fred H. Gage, Salk Institute for Biological Studies
Lawrence S.B. Goldstein, Howard Hughes Medical Institute and University of California, San Diego
Bernard Lo, University of California, San Francisco
Geoffrey Lomax, California Institute for Regenerative Medicine
Gail R. Martin, University of California, San Francisco
P. Pearl O'Rourke, Partners HealthCare System, Inc., and Harvard Medical School
Steven Peckman, University of California, Los Angeles

Janet D. Rowley, University of Chicago
Huda Y. Zoghbi, Howard Hughes Medical Institute and Baylor College of Medicine

Although the reviewers listed above have provided many constructive comments and suggestions, they were not asked to endorse the conclusions or recommendations, nor did they see the final draft of the report before its release. The review of this report was overseen by **Floyd E. Bloom,** The Scripps Research Institute. Appointed by the National Research Council, he was responsible for making certain that an independent examination of this report was carried out in accordance with institutional procedures and that all review comments were carefully considered. Responsibility for the final content of this report rests entirely with the authoring committee and the institution.

Contents

FINAL REPORT OF THE NATIONAL ACADEMIES' HUMAN EMBRYONIC STEM CELL RESEARCH ADVISORY COMMITTEE AND 2010 AMENDMENTS TO THE NATIONAL ACADEMIES' GUIDELINES FOR HUMAN EMBRYONIC STEM CELL RESEARCH

INTRODUCTION

The 2005 National Academies' *Guidelines for Human Embryonic Stem Cell Research* laid out standards for responsible and ethical conduct in a controversial field of research that largely lacked federal funding or oversight. Those guidelines helped this important field of research to develop within a framework of defensible, self-imposed rules. The result was greater public confidence in the quality of the work. As certain states (California, Connecticut, Massachusetts, New York, Maryland, and others) have moved to regulate or fund this research, they have used the National Academies' Guidelines as a template on which to build their own state regulations. The international voluntary standards written by the International Society for Stem Cell Research (ISSCR) also tracked closely the National Academies' Guidelines.

Since their release, the National Academies' Guidelines have been adopted wholly or in large part by most major research institutions in the United States. This response included the creation of new Embryonic Stem Cell Research Oversight (ESCRO) committees, use of detailed guidance on informing gamete and embryo donors, and substantive limitations on the range of materials that would be used and how those experiments would be conducted. To assist the research community, the National Academies' Human Embryonic Stem Cell Research Advisory Committee has conducted regional and other outreach meetings to help investigators and ESCRO committee members to interpret and implement the Guidelines. The Advisory Committee also updated the Guidelines in 2007 and 2008 to reflect the lessons learned by scientists and administrators around the country and to reflect changes in the science of stem cell research. Finally, the Advisory Committee organized or participated in several public workshops on key areas of concern, such as the medical risks of oocyte donation and the next steps toward translating bench science to clinical trials.

The inauguration of President Barack Obama in January 2009 led to a marked shift in federal policies on stem cell research. On March 9, President Obama issued Executive Order (EO) 13505, "Removing Barriers to Responsible Scientific Research Involving Human Stem Cells." (Federal Register Volume 74, Number 46, pp. 10667-10668). President Obama's EO stated that the "Secretary of Health and Human Services, through the Director of NIH [National Institutes of Health], may support and conduct responsible, scientifically worthy human stem cell research, including human embryonic stem cell research, to the extent permitted by law." While leaving untouched the "Dickey-Wicker" amendment,[1] which can only be changed by Congress and which effectively prohibits the use of federal funds to derive new human embryonic stem (hES) cell lines, the EO did rescind prior Executive branch policy. Specifically, the EO rescinded the previous policy that had restricted federal funding for hES cell research to *in vitro* work on lines derived before an earlier EO issued by President George W. Bush, by stating "The Presidential statement of August 9, 2001, limiting Federal funding for research involving human embryonic stem cells, shall have no further effect as a statement of governmental policy."

The EO issued by President Obama also called upon NIH to review its own existing guidance as well as other widely recognized guidelines on human stem cell research, including provisions establishing appropriate safeguards, and to develop and issue new NIH guidance for such research that is consistent with the EO's call to support "responsible, scientifically worthy" stem cell research. Without the restrictions placed upon it by the previous administration, the NIH announced that it would begin a broader

[1] The so-called "Dickey Wicker" amendment has been included in the annual federal appropriation for government-funded activities and has been interpreted to prevent the creation of new human embryonic stem cell lines using federal funds. For example, Section 509 of the Omnibus Appropriations Act 2009, enacted as Public Law 111-8) says:

> None of the funds made available in this Act may be used for—(1) the creation of a human embryo or embryos for research purposes; or (2) research in which a human embryo or embryos are destroyed, discarded, or knowingly subjected to risk of injury or death greater than that allowed for research on fetuses in utero under 45 CFE 46.204(b) and section 498(b) of the Public Health Service Act (42 U.S.C. 289g(b)).

program of funding extramural hES cell research according to its own new guidelines on eligibility for funding.

The NIH Guidelines on Human Stem Cell Research were issued on July 7, 2009 (Appendix A). They establish mechanisms to determine the eligibility of hES cell lines for federal research funding based on the principles that (1) responsible research with hES cells has the potential to improve our understanding of human health and illness and discover new ways to prevent and/or treat illness; and (2) individuals donating embryos for research purposes should do so freely, with voluntary and informed consent. Many of the provisions defining informed consent in the NIH guidelines closely resemble those of the National Academies, ISSCR, and others that predate the new NIH requirements. Thus, the NIH guidelines address both the evaluation of lines already in existence, derived under a variety of rules and guidelines, as well as lines yet to be derived. NIH has established a Working Group of the Advisory Committee to the Director of NIH to determine which hES cell lines were derived under conditions that meet the requirements of the NIH guidelines.[2]

It should be noted that the NIH guidelines prohibit the use of federal funding for research using hES cell lines derived from any source other than excess *in vitro* fertilization (IVF) embryos created for reproductive purposes. Thus research on lines that may, in the future, be derived by somatic cell nuclear transfer (SCNT), parthenogenesis, or from IVF embryos created specifically for research purposes is not currently eligible for federal funding. As a consequence, they would not be subject to the NIH guidelines, including its standards for ensuring voluntary, informed consent for donated materials.

The NIH has also established a new Registry of hES cell lines eligible for NIH funding, containing those lines that its Working Group deems to conform with the requirements of the guidelines.[3] The NIH approved the first list of hES cell lines for NIH funding on December 2, 2009, a second set on December 14, 2009, and additional lines in the first half of 2010 and indicated that it anticipated a continuing flow of approved hES cell lines to be listed on the NIH Registry. Use of those lines with federal funding will henceforth be governed by the NIH guidelines.

This letter report sets out an updated version of the National Academies' Guidelines, one that takes into account the new, expanded role of the NIH in overseeing hES cell research. It also identifies those avenues of continuing National Academies' involvement deemed most valuable by the research community and other significant stakeholders.

---

[2] See <http://www.nih.gov/news/health/sep2009/od-21.htm> for information about the Working Group.

[3] The Registry is available at <http://grants.nih.gov/stem_cells/registry/current.htm>.

THE 2010 NATIONAL ACADEMIES' GUIDELINES

Overall, there are three areas in which non-NIH guidelines will continue to be the source of guidance for hES cell research.

- First, because the continuing effect of the Dickey-Wicker amendment means that derivation of hES cell lines cannot be supported by federal funds, such derivations will need continuing oversight outside the NIH guidelines. And since the acceptability of the cell lines for use in NIH-funded research hinges on the underlying conditions of non-federally funded derivation, the NIH guidelines implicitly overlap many of the National Academies' Guidelines on derivation.

- Second, only hES cell lines derived from excess IVF embryos initially produced for reproductive purposes are currently eligible for NIH funding. Therefore, hES cell lines derived from other sources (e.g., from embryos produced by IVF for research purposes or by nuclear transfer or other methods) will not be eligible for NIH funding and not subject to the NIH guidelines; this work will continue to need oversight under other guidelines.

- Third, because the NIH guidelines only briefly address limits on the research uses to which embryonic stem cell lines may be put, other guidelines will continue to be useful for a wider range of experiments with chimeras than those currently identified by NIH.

To avoid complications, contradictions, and confusion, this Advisory Committee has developed an updated version of the National Academies' Guidelines that recognizes the new and increased influence of the NIH guidelines, and which incorporates references to the NIH guidelines as appropriate in the text of the National Academies' Guidelines. Where there is complete overlap, the Advisory Committee recommends that the NIH guidelines supersede its own. Where there are gaps or limitations in the NIH guidelines, the Advisory Committee recommends continued adoption of its own Guidelines.

The Advisory Committee also notes some areas in which there is tension between NIH, National Academies, and other guidelines or state funding rules, and identifies those for which some variation from National Academies' Guidelines is to be expected.

The first concerns the issue of egg donation. Since the issuance of the 2008 Amendments to the National Academies' Guidelines, the Ethics Committee of the State of New York's Empire State Stem Cell Board adopted a resolution allowing New York State-funded stem cell researchers to compensate women who donate their oocytes directly and solely to research for the time, risk and burden involved in donating.[4] Amounts of compensation are to be comparable to those received by women in New York State for similar donations for reproductive purposes. Compensation may not be based upon number or quality of eggs, but should cover only time and burden. While this Advisory Committee acknowledges that the circumstances surrounding the issue of compensation to oocyte donors continues to evolve, it chose not to change the National Academies' Guidelines. Therefore, the Advisory Committee leaves intact the wording of Section 3.4(b), recognizing that states and other entities may choose to set their own policies, as New York has done.

Second, the Advisory Committee notes that the requirement in the National Academies' Guidelines for consent of *all* gamete donors (see Section 3.3) is not reflected in the new NIH guidelines. Further, a number of states and research institutions have declined to adopt this rule, given the lack of clear legal need for such consent from anonymous donors. The Advisory Committee also notes that the Food and Drug Administration's (FDA's) recent tissue transplant rules require screening of gamete donors except in cases involving sexually intimate partners. This suggests that stem cell lines made with donor (i.e., screened) gametes may be marginally safer for tissue transplants and may be more useable for FDA-regulated trials and therapies. The Advisory Committee recognizes that this requirement may be widely overlooked, and that the issue will be relevant only for a small percentage of derivations. Nonetheless, the Advisory Committee still believes that the practice of obtaining informed consent from all gamete donors, as well as other relevant parties (e.g., intended parents), should continue to be followed because it is the most cautious and respectful standard for donation.

The combination of the new NIH guidelines and those National Academies' Guidelines remaining in effect will continue to represent a comprehensive and responsible approach as this research advances into the future.

THE FUTURE ROLE OF THE NATIONAL ACADEMIES IN STEM CELL RESEARCH OVERSIGHT

In addition to reviewing the National Academies' Guidelines, the Advisory Committee also considered the future role of the National Academies

[4] The resolution is available at <http://stemcell.ny.gov/docs/Compensation_of_Gamete_Donors_resolution_of_Funding_Comm.pdf>

in helping to guide responsible conduct in this field. The Advisory Committee dedicated most of its August 7, 2009, meeting to hear input from stakeholders from the stem cell research community and from those who have experience with the implementation of the National Academies' Guidelines; a list of these individuals participating in the meeting may be found in Appendix B.

One area of considerable discussion was the future of ESCRO committees, as most institutions that have been following the National Academies' or other non-federal guidelines since 2005 have established such committees. Most participants in the August 7 meeting thought that ESCRO/SCRO committees[5] play valuable roles and function in such a way that their elimination could leave gaps not filled by other oversight bodies (e.g., Institutional Review Boards, Institutional Animal Care and Use Committees, Institutional Biosafety Committees). It was stated that ESCRO committees could continue to be useful in maintaining deeper expertise on stem cell research than is necessarily provided by these other oversight bodies. ESCRO committees could also be helpful in assisting research institutions in monitoring developments in the field of stem cell research. In light of these comments, the Advisory Committee agrees that the continued use of ESCRO committees is useful, especially in circumstances where new hES cells are being derived. Even for research with existing cell lines funded by NIH—and therefore subject to NIH guidelines and the NIH hES cell registry—ESCRO committees could also help institutions by providing needed expertise and training for the members of their other committees.

The stakeholders at the August 2009 meeting also discussed whether the National Academies should continue to play a role by maintaining an activity, such as a roundtable, that would allow periodic meetings to discuss knowledge and policy gaps, new problems, and contentious issues. It was suggested that, in the future, the *uses* of stem cells, as opposed to derivation of new lines, are likely to provide a larger share of any controversy or concern surrounding stem cell research. Stakeholders at the meeting suggested that the National Academies are viewed as providing a neutral setting for discussions that can help guide research institutions to make appropriate decisions about research, particularly in areas that are outside the bounds of NIH funding. Several guests stated that research using chimeras represents one such area of potential concern, but that other issues (e.g., stem cell-derived gametes) are also likely to emerge that may provoke controversy. Other topics identified as being potentially important in the future for stem

[5] Other guidelines called for the establishment of Stem Cell Research Oversight (SCRO) committees whose mandate was not limited to *embryonic* stem cell research.

cell research guidance included the relative merits of hES cells vs. induced pluripotent stem cells and clinical trials and translational research.

Some of these topics may have little to do with the Guidelines themselves, but might make excellent topics for future workshops or studies. In light of these discussions, the Advisory Committee decided that:

- The Human Embryonic Stem Cell Research Advisory Committee should prepare this brief final report communicating to the stem cell research community those elements of the National Academies' Guidelines that should remain in effect and under what conditions.

- Following the completion of this task, the Advisory Committee should disband.

The Advisory Committee also discussed the feedback from stakeholders on future mechanisms for discussion of stem cell issues. Although government agencies such as the NIH, professional societies such as the ISSCR, consortia such as the Interstate Alliance on Stem Cell Research,[6] and meetings organized by many different organizations and institutions provide opportunities for discussion, there does not seem to be an ongoing neutral forum for productive discussion of stem cell issues. Participants at the committee's August 2009 meeting mentioned that the National Academies and the Advisory Committee had served this important convening function over the last several years, and there was a need for a similar continuing activity. Perhaps most needed is a forum that could bring together key stakeholders—including federal, state, academic, patient, and industry organizations and institutions— for periodic meetings that would address topics of shared interest and concern to the broader stem cell research, regenerative medicine, and policy communities.

2010 AMENDMENTS TO THE NATIONAL ACADEMIES' GUIDELINES FOR HUMAN EMBRYONIC STEM CELL RESEARCH

Finally, the Advisory Committee presents here an amended version of the National Academies' Guidelines (Appendix C) delineating those sections of the Guidelines that are superseded by the NIH rules for federally funded research.

[6] The Interstate Alliance (IASCR) is a voluntary body of states and affiliate countries and organizations interested in increasing opportunities for interstate collaboration on stem cell research. See <http://www.iascr.org/> for more information.

Appendix A

National Institutes of Health Guidelines for Research Using Human Stem Cells[1]

I. Scope of Guidelines

These Guidelines apply to the expenditure of National Institutes of Health (NIH) funds for research using human embryonic stem cells (hESCs) and certain uses of induced pluripotent stem cells (See Section IV). The Guidelines implement Executive Order 13505.

Long-standing HHS [Department of Health and Human Services] regulations for Protection of Human Subjects, 45 C.F.R. 46, Subpart A establish safeguards for individuals who are the sources of many human tissues used in research, including non-embryonic human adult stem cells and human induced pluripotent stem cells. When research involving human adult stem cells or induced pluripotent stem cells constitutes human subject research, Institutional Review Board review may be required and informed consent may need to be obtained per the requirements detailed in 45 C.F.R. 46, Subpart A. Applicants should consult *http://www.hhs.gov/ohrp/humansubjects/guidance/45cfr46.htm*.

It is also important to note that the HHS regulation, Protection of Human Subjects, 45 C.F.R. Part 46, Subpart A, may apply to certain research using hESCs. This regulation applies, among other things, to research involving individually identifiable private information about a living

[1] Available at <http://stemcells.nih.gov/policy/2009guidelines.htm>.

individual, 45 C.F.R. § 46.102(f). The HHS Office for Human Research Protections (OHRP) considers biological material, such as cells derived from human embryos, to be individually identifiable when they can be linked to specific living individuals by the investigators either directly or indirectly through coding systems. Thus, in certain circumstances, IRB review may be required, in addition to compliance with these Guidelines. Applicant institutions are urged to consult OHRP guidances at *http://www.hhs.gov/ohrp/policy/index.html#topics.*

To ensure that the greatest number of responsibly derived hESCs are eligible for research using NIH funding, these Guidelines are divided into several sections, which apply specifically to embryos donated in the U.S. and foreign countries, both before and on or after the effective date of these Guidelines. Section II (A) and (B) describe the conditions and review processes for determining hESC eligibility for NIH funds. Further information on these review processes may be found at *www.NIH.gov.* Sections IV and V describe research that is not eligible for NIH funding.

These guidelines are based on the following principles:

1. Responsible research with hESCs has the potential to improve our understanding of human health and illness and discover new ways to prevent and/or treat illness.
2. Individuals donating embryos for research purposes should do so freely, with voluntary and informed consent.

As directed by Executive Order 13505, the NIH shall review and update these Guidelines periodically, as appropriate.

II. Eligibility of Human Embryonic Stem Cells for Research with NIH Funding

For the purpose of these Guidelines, "human embryonic stem cells (hESCs)" are cells that are derived from the inner cell mass of blastocyst stage human embryos, are capable of dividing without differentiating for a prolonged period in culture, and are known to develop into cells and tissues of the three primary germ layers.[2] Although hESCs are derived from embryos, such stem cells are not themselves human embryos. All of the processes and procedures for review of the eligibility of hESCs will be centralized at the NIH as follows:

A. Applicant institutions proposing research using hESCs derived from embryos donated in the U.S. on or after the effective date of these Guidelines may use hESCs that are posted on the new NIH Registry or they may establish eligibility for NIH funding by submitting an assurance of compliance with Section II (A) of the Guidelines, along with supporting information demonstrating compliance for administrative review by the NIH. For the purposes of this Section II (A), hESCs should have been derived from human embryos:
   1. that were created using in vitro fertilization for reproductive purposes and were no longer needed for this purpose;
   2. that were donated by individuals who sought reproductive treatment (hereafter referred to as "donor(s)") and who gave voluntary written consent for the human embryos to be used for research purposes; and
   3. for which all of the following can be assured and documentation provided, such as consent forms, written policies, or other documentation, provided:
      a. All options available in the health care facility where treatment was sought pertaining to the embryos no longer needed for reproductive purposes were explained to the individual(s) who sought reproductive treatment.
      b. No payments, cash or in kind, were offered for the donated embryos.
      c. Policies and/or procedures were in place at the health care facility where the embryos were donated that neither consenting nor refusing to donate embryos for research would affect the quality of care provided to potential donor(s).

---

[2] On February 23, 2010, NIH issued a request for public comment in the Federal Register on changing this definition to the following:

> For the Purpose of the Guidelines, 'human embryonic stem cells (hESCs)' are pluripotent cells that are derived from early stage human embryos, up to and including the blastocyst stage, are capable of dividing without differentiating for a prolonged period in culture, and are known to develop into cells and tissues of the three primary germ layers.

As of the publication of this report, no revisions have been formally issued. Readers are encouraged to consult <http://stemcells.nih.gov/> for the NIH current guidelines.

d. There was a clear separation between the prospective donor(s)'s decision to create human embryos for reproductive purposes and the prospective donor(s)'s decision to donate human embryos for research purposes. Specifically:
   i. Decisions related to the creation of human embryos for reproductive purposes should have been made free from the influence of researchers proposing to derive or utilize hESCs in research. The attending physician responsible for reproductive clinical care and the researcher deriving and/or proposing to utilize hESCs should not have been the same person unless separation was not practicable.
   ii. At the time of donation, consent for that donation should have been obtained from the individual(s) who had sought reproductive treatment. That is, even if potential donor(s) had given prior indication of their intent to donate to research any embryos that remained after reproductive treatment, consent for the donation for research purposes should have been given at the time of the donation.
   iii. Donor(s) should have been informed that they retained the right to withdraw consent for the donation of the embryo until the embryos were actually used to derive embryonic stem cells or until information which could link the identity of the donor(s) with the embryo was no longer retained, if applicable.

e. During the consent process, the donor(s) were informed of the following:
   i. that the embryos would be used to derive hESCs for research;
   ii. what would happen to the embryos in the derivation of hESCs for research;
   iii. that hESCs derived from the embryos might be kept for many years;
   iv. that the donation was made without any restriction or direction regarding the individual(s) who may receive medical benefit from the use of the hESCs, such as who may be the recipients of cell transplants.;
   v. that the research was not intended to provide direct medical benefit to the donor(s);

vi. that the results of research using the hESCs may have commercial potential, and that the donor(s) would not receive financial or any other benefits from any such commercial development;

vii. whether information that could identify the donor(s) would be available to researchers.

B. Applicant institutions proposing research using hESCs derived from embryos donated in the U.S. before the effective date of these Guidelines may use hESCs that are posted on the new NIH Registry or they may establish eligibility for NIH funding in one of two ways:

1. By complying with Section II (A) of the Guidelines; or
2. By submitting materials to a Working Group of the Advisory Committee to the Director (ACD), which will make recommendations regarding eligibility for NIH funding to its parent group, the ACD. The ACD will make recommendations to the NIH Director, who will make final decisions about eligibility for NIH funding.

   The materials submitted must demonstrate that the hESCs were derived from human embryos: 1) that were created using in vitro fertilization for reproductive purposes and were no longer needed for this purpose; and 2) that were donated by donor(s) who gave voluntary written consent for the human embryos to be used for research purposes.

   The Working Group will review submitted materials, e.g., consent forms, written policies or other documentation, taking into account the principles articulated in Section II (A), 45 C.F.R. Part 46, Subpart A, and the following additional points to consider. That is, during the informed consent process, including written or oral communications, whether the donor(s) were: (1) informed of other available options pertaining to the use of the embryos; (2) offered any inducements for the donation of the embryos; and (3) informed about what would happen to the embryos after the donation for research.

C. For embryos donated outside the United States before the effective date of these Guidelines, applicants may comply with either Section II (A) or (B). For embryos donated outside of the United States on or after the effective date of the Guidelines, applicants seeking to determine eligibility for NIH research funding may submit an assurance that the hESCs fully comply with Section II (A) or submit an assurance along with supporting information, that the alternative procedural standards of the foreign country where the embryo was donated provide protections at least equivalent to those provided by Section II (A) of these Guidelines. These materials will be reviewed by the NIH ACD Working Group, which will recommend to the ACD whether such equivalence exists. Final decisions will be made by the NIH Director.

D. NIH will establish a new Registry listing hESCs eligible for use in NIH funded research. All hESCs that have been reviewed and deemed eligible by the NIH in accordance with these Guidelines will be posted on the new NIH Registry.

III. Use of NIH Funds

Prior to the use of NIH funds, funding recipients should provide assurances, when endorsing applications and progress reports submitted to NIH for projects using hESCs, that the hESCs are listed on the NIH registry.

IV. Research Using hESCs and/or Human Induced Pluripotent Stem Cells That, Although the Cells May Come from Eligible Sources, Is Nevertheless Ineligible for NIH Funding

This section governs research using hESCs and human induced pluripotent stem cells, i.e., human cells that are capable of dividing without differentiating for a prolonged period in culture, and are known to develop into cells and tissues of the three primary germ layers. Although the cells may come from eligible sources, the following uses of these cells are nevertheless ineligible for NIH funding, as follows:

A. Research in which hESCs (even if derived from embryos donated in accordance with these Guidelines) or human induced pluripotent stem cells are introduced into non-human primate blastocysts.
B. Research involving the breeding of animals where the introduction of hESCs (even if derived from embryos donated in accordance with these Guidelines) or human induced pluripotent stem cells may contribute to the germ line.

V. Other Research Not Eligible for NIH Funding

A. NIH funding of the derivation of stem cells from human embryos is prohibited by the annual appropriations ban on funding of human embryo research (Section 509, Omnibus Appropriations Act, 2009, Pub. L. 111-8, 3/11/09), otherwise known as the Dickey Amendment.

B. Research using hESCs derived from other sources, including somatic cell nuclear transfer, parthenogenesis, and/or IVF embryos created for research purposes, is not eligible for NIH funding.

Appendix B

Invited Participants at the August 7, 2009, Meeting of the Human Embryonic Stem Cell Research Advisory Committee

GEORGE Q. DALEY, Samuel E. Lux IV Chair in Hematology and Director, Stem Cell Transplantation Program, Children's Hospital Boston; Associate Professor of Biological Chemistry and Molecular Pharmacology, Harvard Medical School; Investigator, Howard Hughes Medical Institute; and Past President, International Society for Stem Cell Research

DEBORAH A. HURSH, Senior Investigator, Division of Cellular and Gene Therapies, Center for Biologics Research and Review, U.S. Food and Drug Administration

JULIE KANESHIRO, Team Leader, Policy, Office for Human Research Protections, Department of Health and Human Services

STORY LANDIS, Director, National Institute of Neurological Disorders and Stroke, National Institutes of Health (NIH), and Chair, NIH Stem Cell Task Force

BERNARD LO, Professor of Medicine and Director of the Program in Medical Ethics, University of California, San Francisco

GEOFF LOMAX, Senior Officer to the Standards Working Group, California Institute for Regenerative Medicine

JOHN MCNEISH, Executive Director, Pfizer Regenerative Medicine

P. PEARL O'ROURKE, Director of Human Research Affairs, Partners HealthCare System, Boston; and Associate Professor of Pediatrics, Harvard Medical School

SEAN TIPTON, Past-President, Coalition for the Advancement of Medical Research; and Director of Public Affairs, American Society for Reproductive Medicine

Appendix C

National Academies' Guidelines for Human Embryonic Stem Cell Research Amended as of May 2010[7]

1.0 Introduction
2.0 Establishment of an Institutional Embryonic Stem Cell Research Oversight Committee
3.0 Procurement of Gametes, Morulae, Blastocysts or Cells for Generation of hES ~~Generation~~ Cell Lines
4.0 Derivation of hES Cell Lines
5.0 Banking and Distribution of hES Cell Lines
6.0 Research Use of hES Cell Lines
7.0 International Collaboration
8.0 Conclusion

1.0 INTRODUCTION

~~In this chapter we collect all the recommendations made throughout the report and translate them into a series of formal guidelines.~~ These guidelines focus on the derivation, procurement, banking, and use of human embryonic stem (hES) cell lines and some uses of human pluripotent (hPS) cell lines. They provide an oversight process that will help to ensure that research with hES cells is conducted in a responsible and ethically sensitive manner and in compliance with all regulatory requirements pertaining to biomedical research in general. The National Academies ~~are issuing~~ issues these guidelines

[7] New or modified wording is indicated by underlining. Deleted wording is indicated by ~~strikethrough~~.

for the use of the scientific community, including researchers in university, industry, or other private-sector research organizations who are conducting such research with non-federal funding. Researchers conducting federally-funded hES cell research should, however, note that the requirements of the National Institutes of Health (NIH)—available at http://stemcells.nih.gov/policy/2009guidelines.htm—supersede these National Academies' Guidelines for certain sections (as noted below).

1.1 What These Guidelines Cover

1.1(a) These guidelines cover all derivation of hES cell lines and all research that uses hES cells derived from

- (i) blastocysts and/or morulae made for reproductive purposes and later obtained for research from *in vitro* fertilization (IVF) clinics,
- (ii) blastocysts and/or morulae made specifically for research using IVF,
- (iii) somatic cell nuclear transfer (NT) into oocytes or by parthenogensis or androgenesis.

1.1(b) Some of the concerns addressed in this report are common to other types of human stem cell research; as such, certain of these Guidelines should also apply to those other types of research. For example,

- (i) research that uses human adult stem cells,
- (ii) research that uses fetal stem cells or embryonic germ cells derived from fetal tissue; such research is covered by federal statutory restrictions at 42 U.S.C. 289g-2(a) and federal regulations at 45 CFR 46.210,
- (iii) research using hPS cells derived from non-embryonic sources, such as spermatogonial stem cells and "induced pluripotent" stem cells derived from somatic cells by introduction of genes or otherwise (so-called iPS cells), as well as other pluripotent cells yet to be developed; guidelines for hPS cells are collected in Section 7 below.

~~Recommendations as to which guidelines apply to other hPS cells are collected in a new Section 7 below. Institutions and investigators conducting research with adult and fetal stem cells should also consider which individual provisions of these guidelines are relevant to their research.~~

1.1(c) Research supported by NIH funds using NIH-approved hES cell lines is governed by NIH guidelines.

1.1(d) The guidelines do not cover research that uses nonhuman stem cells.

1.2 Reproductive Uses of NT

These guidelines also do not apply to reproductive uses of nuclear transfer, which are addressed in the 2002 report *Scientific and Medical Aspects of Human Reproductive Cloning*, in which the National Academies recommended that "Human reproductive cloning should not now be practiced. It is dangerous and likely to fail." Although these guidelines do not specifically address human reproductive cloning, it continues to be the view of the National Academies that research aimed at the reproductive cloning of a human being should not be conducted at this time.

1.3 Categories of hES Cell Research

These guidelines specify categories of research that:

- Are permissible after currently mandated reviews and proper notification of the relevant research institution.
- Are permissible after additional review by an Embryonic Stem Cell Research Oversight (ESCRO) committee, as described in Section 2.0 of the guidelines.
- Should not be conducted at this time.

Because of the sensitive nature of some aspects of hES cell research, these guidelines in many instances set a higher standard than is required by laws or regulations with which institutions and individuals already must comply.

1.3(a) hES Cell Research Permissible after Currently Mandated Reviews

Purely *in vitro* hES cell research that uses previously derived hES cell lines is permissible provided that the ESCRO committee or equivalent body designated by the investigator's institution (see Section 2.0) receives documentation of the provenance of the cell lines including (i) documentation of the use of an acceptable informed consent process that was approved by an Institutional Review Board (IRB) or foreign equivalent for their derivation (consistent with Section 3.6) and (ii) documentation of compliance with ~~any~~

~~additional required review by~~ an Institutional Animal Care and Use Committee (IACUC), Institutional Biosafety Committee (IBC), or other institutionally mandated review, if necessary. To determine whether the proposed research meets the requirements of this section, the ESCRO committee may choose to conduct an "expedited review" of such research proposals. In this context, *expedited review* means that the ESCRO committee chair or others designated by the committee chair act on behalf of the committee to determine that the hES cells have been acceptably derived (see Section 1.5) and report to the entire committee. All hES cell lines listed on the NIH Registry of approved lines are acceptable for use in research, subject to any restrictions imposed by NIH. Certain other lines may be considered acceptable for research using non-federal funds (see 1.5 below).

1.3(b) hES Cell Research Permissible Only After Additional Review and Approval

(i) Generation of new lines of hES cells by whatever means.

(ii) Research involving the introduction of hES cells into ~~non-human~~ animals other than humans or primates[8] at any stage of embryonic, fetal, or postnatal development. Particular attention should be paid to at least three factors: the extent to which the implanted cells colonize and integrate into the animal tissue; the degree of differentiation of the implanted cells; and the possible effects of the implanted cells on the function of the animal tissue.

(iii) Research involving the introduction of hES cell into nonhuman primates at any stage of fetal or postnatal development. Particular attention should be paid to at least three factors: the extent to which the implanted cells colonize and integrate into the animal tissue; the degree of differentiation of the implanted cells; and the possible effects of the implanted cells on the function of the animal tissue.

(iv) Research in which the identity of the donors of blastocysts, morulae, gametes, or somatic cells from which the hES cells were derived is readily ascertainable or might become known to the investigator.

---

[8] "Nonhuman animals" has been changed to "animals other than human or primates" as the Guidelines do not permit the introduction of hES cells into humans or nonhuman primates (Section 1.3(c)(ii)).

1.3(c) hES Cell Research That Should Not Be Permitted At This Time

The following types of research should not be conducted at this time:

(i) Research involving *in vitro* culture of any intact human embryo, regardless of derivation method, for longer than 14 days or until formation of the primitive streak begins, whichever occurs first.

(ii) Research in which hES cells are introduced into nonhuman primate blastocysts or in which any embryonic stem cells are introduced into human blastocysts.

In addition:

(iii) No animal into which hES cells have been introduced such that they could contribute to the germ line should be allowed to breed.

1.4 Obligations of Investigators and Institutions

All scientific investigators and their institutions, regardless of their field, bear the ultimate responsibility for ensuring that they conduct themselves in accordance with professional standards and with integrity. In particular, people whose research involves hES cells should work closely with oversight bodies, demonstrate respect for the autonomy and privacy of those who donate gametes, morulae, blastocysts, or somatic cells and be sensitive to public concerns about research that involves human embryos.

~~1.5 Use of NIH-approved hES cell lines~~

~~1.5(a) It is acceptable to use hES cell lines that were approved in August 2001 for use in U.S. federally funded research.~~

~~1.5(b) ESCRO committees should include on their registry a list of NIH-approved cell lines that have been used at their institution in accord with the requirement in section 2.0 of the Guidelines.~~

~~1.5(c) Presence on the list of NIH-approved cell lines constitutes adequate documentation of provenance, as per Section 6.1 of the Guidelines.~~

1.5 Acceptability of research using hES cell lines imported from other institutions or jurisdictions

1.5(a) Before approving use of hES ~~and hPS~~ cell lines imported from other institutions or jurisdictions, ESCRO committees should consider whether such cell lines have been "acceptably derived."

1.5(b) "Acceptably derived" means that the cell lines were derived from gametes or embryos for which

- (i) the donation protocol was reviewed and approved by an IRB or, in the case of donations taking place outside the United States, a substantially equivalent oversight body;
- (ii) consent to donate was voluntary and informed;
- (iii) donation was made with reimbursement policies consistent with these Guidelines; and
- (iv) donation and derivation complied with the extant legal requirements of the relevant jurisdiction.

1.5(c) ESCRO committees should include on their registry a list of cell lines that have been imported from other institutions or jurisdictions and information on the specific guidelines, regulations, or statutes under which the derivation of the imported cell lines was conducted. This is in accord with the requirement in section 2.0 of the Guidelines that calls for ESCRO committees to maintain registries listing the cell lines in use at their institutions.

2.0 ESTABLISHMENT OF AN INSTITUTIONAL EMBRYONIC STEM CELL RESEARCH OVERSIGHT COMMITTEE

To provide oversight of all issues related to derivation and use of hES cell lines and to facilitate education of investigators involved in hES cell research, ~~each~~ many institutions currently require that research ~~should have activities~~ involving hES cells should be overseen by an Embryonic Stem Cell Research Oversight (ESCRO) committee. Although not required under the NIH Guidelines on Human Stem Cell Research, institutions conducting federally funded stem cell research are nevertheless likely to decide to maintain their ESCRO committees and use them for consultation, training, and any other functions appropriate to assist the institution and its researchers in evaluating and managing hES cell research. Institutions that conduct both federally funded and non-federally funded hES cell research, particularly if this research involves the derivation of new cell lines, should maintain and use their ESCRO committees as they did prior to July 7, 2009. An ESCRO committee could be internal to a single institution or established jointly with one or more other institutions. Alternatively, an institution may have its proposals reviewed by an ESCRO committee of another institution, or by an independent ESCRO committee. An ESCRO committee should include independent representatives of the lay public as well as persons with expertise in developmental biology, stem cell research, molecular biology, assisted reproduction, and ethical and legal issues in hES cell research. It must have suitable scientific, medical, and ethical expertise to conduct its own review and should have the resources needed to coordinate the management of the various other reviews required for a particular protocol. A pre-existing committee could serve the functions of the ESCRO committee provided that it has the expertise recommended here and representation to perform the various roles described in this report. For example, an institution might elect to constitute an ESCRO committee from among some members of an IRB. But the ESCRO committee should not be a subcommittee of the IRB, as its responsibilities extend beyond human subject protections. Furthermore, much hES cell research does not require IRB review. The ESCRO committee ~~should~~ would:

- (a) Provide oversight over all issues related to derivation ~~and use~~ of hES cell lines.
- (b) Provide oversight over issues related to the use of hES cell lines not otherwise covered by NIH guidelines.
- (~~b~~c) Review and approve the scientific merit of research protocols.
- (~~c~~d) Review compliance of all in-house hES cell research with all relevant regulations and these guidelines.
- (~~d~~e) Maintain registries of hES cell research conducted at the institution and hES cell lines derived or imported by institutional investigators. An institution conducting stem cell research should make information from the registries (including, but not necessarily limited to, project abstracts and source of funding) available to the public and the media through the institution's Web site.
- (~~e~~f) Facilitate education of investigators involved in hES cell research.

An institution that maintains its own ESCRO committee should also conduct periodic audits of the committee to verify that it is carrying out its responsibilities appropriately. Auditable records include documentation of decisions regarding the acceptability of research proposals and verification that cell lines in use at the institution were acceptably derived (see Section 1.5). Institutions should make the results of these audits available to the public.

An institution that uses an external ESCRO committee should nevertheless ensure that the registry and educational functions of an internal ESCRO committee are carried out by the external ESCRO committee on its behalf or internally by other administrative units. Institutions that use external ESCRO committees are also responsible for ensuring that these committees are likewise carrying out their responsibilities appropriately.

2.1 For projects that involve more than one institution, review of the scientific merit, justification, and compliance status of the research may be carried out by a single ESCRO committee if all participating institutions agree to accept the results of the review.

3.0 PROCUREMENT OF GAMETES, MORULAE, BLASTOCYSTS OR CELLS FOR GENERATION OF hES CELL LINES ~~GENERATION~~

3.1 An IRB, as described in federal regulations at 45 CFR 46.107, should review all new procurement of all gametes, morulae, blastocysts, or somatic cells for the purpose of generating new hES or hPS cell lines. This includes the procurement of blastocysts and/or morulae in excess of clinical need from infertility clinics, blastocysts made through IVF specifically for research purposes, and oocytes, sperm, and somatic cells donated for development of hES cell lines derived through NT or by parthenogenesis or androgenesis; and hPS cells derived by any means that require human subjects review.

3.2 Consent for donation should be obtained from each donor at the time of donation. Even people who have given prior indication of their intent to donate to research any blastocysts and/or morulae that remain after clinical care should nonetheless give informed consent at the time of donation. Donors should be informed that they retain the right to withdraw consent until the blastocysts and/or morulae are actually used in cell line derivation.

3.3 When donor gametes have been used in the IVF process, resulting blastocysts and/or morulae may not be used for research without consent of all gamete donors. Written agreement at the time of gamete donation that one potential use of the blastocysts and/or morulae is embryo research will constitute sufficient consent.

3.4 Payment and Reimbursement

3.4 (a) No payments, cash or in-kind, may be provided for donating blastocysts and/or morulae in excess of clinical need for research purposes. People who elect to donate stored blastocysts and/or morulae for research should not be reimbursed for the costs of storage prior to the decision to donate.

3.4(b) Women who undergo hormonal induction to generate oocytes specifically for research purposes (such as for NT) should be reimbursed only for direct expenses incurred as a result of the procedure, as determined by an IRB. Direct expenses may include costs associated with travel, housing, child care, medical care, health insurance, and actual lost wages. No payments beyond reimbursements, cash or in-kind, should be provided for donating oocytes for research purposes. Similarly, no payments beyond reimbursements should be made for donations of sperm for research purposes or of somatic cells for use in NT.

3.5 To facilitate autonomous choice, decisions related to the creation of embryos for infertility treatment should be free of the influence of investigators who propose to derive or use hES cells in research. Whenever it is practicable, the attending physician responsible for the infertility treatment and the investigator deriving or proposing to use hES cells should not be the same person.

3.6 In the context of donation of gametes, morulae, blastocysts, or somatic cells for hES cell research or for hPS cell research that requires human subjects review, the informed consent process, should, at a minimum, provide the following information.[9]

(a) A statement that the ~~blastocysts~~, gametes, morulae, blastocysts, or somatic cells will be used to derive hES or hPS cells for research that may include research on human transplantation.

(b) A statement that the donation is made without any restriction or direction regarding who may be the recipient of transplants of the cells derived, except in the case of autologous donation.

(c) A statement as to whether the identities of the donors will be readily ascertainable to those who derive or work with the resulting hES or hPS cell lines.

[9] To be eligible for use in federally-funded research, the NIH guidelines specify specific elements for informed consent that may differ from the elements listed below.

(d) If the identities of the donors are retained (even if coded), a statement as to whether donors wish to be contacted in the future to receive information obtained through studies of the cell lines.
(e) An assurance that participants in research projects will follow applicable and appropriate best practices for donation, procurement, culture, and storage of cells and tissues to ensure, in particular, the traceability of stem cells. (Traceable information, however, must be secured to ensure confidentiality.)
(f) A statement that derived hES or hPS cells and/or cell lines might be kept for many years.
(g) A statement that the hES or hPS cells and/or cell lines might be used in research involving genetic manipulation of the cells or the mixing of human and nonhuman cells in animal models.
(h) Disclosure of the possibility that the results of study of the hES or hPS cells may have commercial potential and a statement that the donor will not receive financial or any other benefits from any future commercial development.
(i) A statement that the research is not intended to provide direct medical benefit to the donor(s) except in the case of autologous donation.
(j) A statement that embryos will be destroyed in the process of deriving hES cells.
(k) A statement that neither consenting nor refusing to donate embryos for research will affect the quality of any future care provided to potential donors.
(l) A statement of the risks involved to the donor.

In addition, donors could be offered the option of agreeing to some forms of hES cell research but not others. For example, donors might agree to have their materials used for deriving new hES cell lines but might not want their materials used, for example, for NT. The consent process should fully explore whether donors have objections to any specific forms of research to ensure that their wishes are honored. Investigators and stem cell banks are, of course, free to choose which cell lines to accept, and are not obligated to accept cell lines for which maintaining information about specific research use prohibitions would be unduly burdensome.

New derivations of stem cell lines from banked tissues obtained prior to the adoption of these guidelines are permissible provided that the original donations were made in accordance with the legal requirements in force at the place and time of donation. This includes gametes, morulae, blastocysts, adult stem cells, somatic cells, or other tissue. In the event that these banked tissues retain identifiers linked to living individuals, human subjects protections may apply.

3.7 Clinical personnel who have a conscientious objection to hES cell research should not be required to participate in providing donor information or securing donor consent for research use of gametes, morulae, or blastocysts. That privilege should not extend to the care of a donor or recipient.

3.8 Researchers may not ask members of the infertility treatment team to generate more oocytes than necessary for the optimal chance of reproductive success. An infertility clinic or other third party responsible for obtaining consent or collecting materials should not be able to pay for or be paid for the material obtained (except for specifically defined cost-based reimbursements and payments for professional services).

4.0 DERIVATION OF hES CELL LINES

4.1 Requests to the ESCRO committee for permission to attempt derivation of new hES cell lines from donated embryos, morulae, or blastocysts must include evidence of IRB approval of the procurement process (see Section 3.0 above).

4.2 The scientific rationale for the need to generate new hES cell lines, by whatever means, must be clearly presented, and the basis for the numbers of embryos, morulae, and blastocysts needed should be justified.

4.3 Research teams should demonstrate appropriate expertise or training in derivation or culture of either human or nonhuman ES cells before permission to derive new lines is given.

4.4 When NT experiments involving either human or nonhuman oocytes are proposed as a route to generation of hES cells, the protocol must have a strong scientific rationale. Proposals that include studies to find alternatives to donated oocytes in this research should be encouraged.

4.5 Neither blastocysts or morulae made using NT of human nuclei (whether produced with human or nonhuman oocytes) nor parthenogenetic or androgenetic human embryos may be transferred to a human or nonhuman uterus or cultured as intact embryos *in vitro* for longer than 14 days or until formation of the primitive streak, whichever occurs first.

4.6 Investigators must document how they will characterize, validate, store, and distribute any new hES cell lines and how they will maintain the confidentiality of any coded or identifiable information associated with the lines (see Section 5.0 below). Investigators are encouraged to apply the same procedures and standards for characterization, validation, storage, and distribution to hPS cell lines.

5.0 BANKING AND DISTRIBUTION OF hES CELL LINES

There are several models for the banking of human biological materials, including hES cells. The most relevant is the U.K. Stem Cell Bank. The guidelines developed by this and other groups generally adhere to key ethical principles that focus on the need for consent of donors and a system for monitoring adherence to ethical, legal, and scientific requirements. As hES cell research advances, it will be increasingly important for institutions that are obtaining, storing, and using cell lines to have confidence in the value of stored cells—that is, that they were obtained ethically and with the informed consent of donors, that they are well characterized and screened for safety, and that the conditions under which they are maintained and stored meet the highest scientific standards. Institutions engaged in hES research should seek mechanisms for establishing central repositories for hES cell lines—through partnerships or augmentation of existing quality research cell line repositories and should adhere to high ethical, legal, and scientific standards. At a minimum, an institutional registry of stem cell lines should be maintained. Institutions are encouraged to consider the use of the same procedures for banking and distribution of hPS cell lines.

5.1 Institutions that are banking or plan to bank hES cell lines should establish uniform guidelines to ensure that donors of material give informed consent through a process approved by an IRB and that meticulous records are maintained about all aspects of cell culture. Uniform tracking systems and common guidelines for distribution of cells should be established.

5.2 Any facility engaged in obtaining and storing hES cell lines should consider the following standards:

(a) Creation of a committee for policy and oversight purposes and creation of clear and standardized protocols for banking and withdrawals.

(b) Documentation requirements for investigators and sites that deposit cell lines, including

(i) A copy of the donor consent form.
(ii) Proof of Institutional Review Board approval of the procurement process.
(iii) Available medical information on the donors, including results of infectious-disease screening.
(iv) Available clinical, observational, or diagnostic information about the donor(s).
(v) Critical information about culture conditions (such as media, cell passage, and safety information).
(vi) Available cell line characterization (such as karyotype and genetic markers).

A repository has the right of refusal if prior culture conditions or other items do not meet its standards.

(c) A secure system for protecting the privacy of donors when materials retain codes or identifiable information, including but not limited to
(i) A schema for maintaining confidentiality (such as a coding system).
(ii) A system for a secure audit trail from primary cell lines to those submitted to the repository.
(iii) A policy governing whether and how to deliver clinically significant information back to donors.

(d) The following standard practices:
(i) Assignment of a unique identifier to each sample.
(ii) A process for characterizing cell lines.
(iii) A process for expanding, maintaining, and storing cell lines.
(iv) A system for quality assurance and control.
(v) A website that contains scientific descriptions and data related to the cell lines available.
(vi) A procedure for reviewing applications for cell lines.
(vii) A process for tracking disbursed cell lines and recording their status when shipped (such as number of passages).
(viii) A system for auditing compliance.
(ix) A schedule of charges.
(x) A statement of intellectual property policies.
(xi) When appropriate, creation of a clear Material Transfer Agreement or user agreement.
(xii) A liability statement.
(xiii) A system for disposal of material.

(e) Clear criteria for distribution of cell lines, including but not limited to evidence of approval of the research by an embryonic stem cell research oversight committee or equivalent body at the recipient institution.

6.0 RESEARCH USE OF hES CELL LINES

Once hES cell lines have been derived, investigators and institutions, through ESCRO committees and other relevant committees (such as an IACUC, an IBC, or a radiation safety committee) should monitor their use in research.

6.1 Institutions should require documentation of the provenance of all hES cell lines, whether the cells were imported into the institution or generated locally. The institution should obtain evidence of IRB-approval of the procurement process and of adherence to basic ethical and legal principles of procurement as described in Section 1.3(a) and 1.5. In the case of lines imported from another institution, documentation that these criteria were met at the time of derivation will suffice. Listing on the NIH Registry will be sufficient evidence of acceptability of hES cell lines.

6.2 *In vitro* experiments involving the use of already derived and coded hES cell lines will not need review beyond the review described in Sections 1.3(a) and 6.1.

6.3 Each institution should maintain a registry of its investigators who are conducting hES cell research and ensure that all registered users are kept up to date with changes in guidelines and regulations regarding the use of hES cells.

6.4 All protocols involving the combination of hES cells with nonhuman embryos, fetuses, or adult vertebrate animals must be submitted to the local IACUC for review of animal welfare issues and to the ESCRO committee for consideration of the consequences of the human contributions to the resulting chimeras. (See also Section 1.3(c)(iii) concerning breeding of chimeras.)

6.5 Transplantation of differentiated derivatives of hES cells or even hES cells themselves into adult animals will not require extensive ESCRO committee review. If there is a possibility that the human cells could contribute in a major organized way to the brain of the recipient animal, however, the scientific justification for the experiments must be strong, and proof of principle using nonhuman (preferably primate) cells, is desirable.

6.6 Experiments in which hES cells, their derivatives, or other pluripotent cells are introduced into nonhuman fetuses and allowed to develop into adult chimeras need more careful consideration because the extent of human contribution to the resulting animal may be higher. Consideration of any major functional contributions to the brain should be a main focus of review. (See also Section 1.3(c)(iii) concerning breeding of chimeras.)

6.7 Introduction of hES cells into nonhuman mammalian blastocysts should be considered only under circumstances in which no other experiment can provide the information needed. (See also Sections 1.3(c)(ii) and 1.3(c)(iii) concerning restrictions on breeding of chimeras and production of chimeras with nonhuman primate blastocysts.)

6.8 Research use of existing hES cells does not require IRB review unless the research involves introduction of the hES cells or their derivatives into patients or the possibility that the identity of the donors of the ~~blastocysts~~, gametes, morulae, blastocysts, or somatic cells is readily ascertainable or might become known to the investigator.

7.0 RECOMMENDATIONS FOR RESEARCH USE OF NON-EMBRYO-DERIVED HUMAN PLURIPOTENT STEM CELLS (hPS CELLS)

7.1 Derivation

Because non-embryo-derived hPS cells are derived from human material, their derivation ~~is~~ may be covered by existing IRB regulations concerning review and informed consent, depending on the source of the tissue used. No ESCRO committee review is necessary, although the IRB may always seek the advice of an ESCRO committee if this seems desirable. Where appropriate, t~~T~~he IRB review should consider proper consent for use of the derived hPS cells. Some of the recommendations for informed consent that apply to hES cells also apply to hPS cells (see Section 3.6), including informed consent to genetic manipulation of resulting pluripotent stem cells and their use for transplantation into animals and humans and potentially in future commercial development.

7.2 Use in *in Vitro* Experiments

Use of hPS cells in purely *in vitro* experiments need not be subject to any review beyond that necessary for any human cell line except that any experiments designed or expected to yield gametes (oocytes or sperm) should be subject to ESCRO committee review.

7.3 Use in Experiments Involving Transplantation of hPS Cells into Animals at any Stage of Development or Maturity

~~7.3(a) Research involving transplantation of pluripotent human cells derived from nonembryonic sources into nonhuman animals other than humans or primates at any stage of embryonic, fetal, or postnatal development should be reviewed by ESCRO committees and IACUCs, as are similar experiments that use hES cells.~~

~~7.3(b) ESCRO committees should review the provenance of the hPS cells as they review the provenance of hES cells (see section 1.5) to ensure that the cell lines were derived according to ethical procedures of informed consent as monitored by an IRB or equivalent oversight body.~~

~~7.3()~~ Proposals for use of hPS cells in animals should be considered in one of the following categories:

(i) Permissible after currently mandated reviews and proper documentation [see Section 1.3(a)]: experiments that are exempt from full ESCRO committee review but not IACUC review (experiments that involve only transplantation into postnatal animals with no likelihood of contributing to the central nervous system or germ line).

(ii) Permissible after additional review by an ESCRO committee, as described in Section 2.0 of the guidelines [see Section 1.3(b)]: experiments in which there is a significant possibility that the implanted hPS cells could give rise to neural or gametic cells and tissues. Such experiments need full ESCRO committee and IACUC review and would include generation of all preimplantation chimeras as well as neural transplantation into embryos or perinatal animals. Particular attention should be paid to at least three factors: the extent to which the implanted cells colonize and integrate into the animal tissue; the degree of differentiation of the implanted cells; and the possible effects of the implanted cells on the function of the animal tissue.

(iii) Should not be conducted at this time [see Section 1.3(c)]

(1) Experiments that involve transplantation of hPS cells into human blastocysts.
(2) Research in which hPS cells are introduced into nonhuman primate embryos, pending further research that will clarify the potential of such introduced cells to contribute to neural tissue or to the germ line.

7.4 Multipotent Neural Stem Cells

It is also relevant to note that neural stem cells, although not pluripotent, are multipotent and may have the potential to contribute to neural tissue in chimeric animals. ESCRO committees should decide whether they wish to review and monitor such experiments with neural stem cells in a similar fashion.

7.5 Prohibition on Breeding

No animal into which hPS cells have been introduced such that they could contribute to the germ line should be allowed to breed.

7.6 Guidance for Banking and Distribution

Institutions should consider the value of banking and distributing hPS cells using the guidance and rules that are already in place for hES cells and the value of including hPS cell lines in their registries.

8.0 INTERNATIONAL COLLABORATION

If a U.S.-based investigator collaborates with an investigator in another country, the ESCRO committee may determine that the procedures prescribed by the foreign institution afford protections consistent with these guidelines, and the ESCRO committee may approve the substitution of some of or all of the foreign procedures for its own.

9.0 CONCLUSION

The substantial public support for hES cell research and the growing trend by many nonfederal funding agencies and state legislatures to support this field requires a set of guidelines to provide a framework for hES cell research. In the absence of the oversight ~~that would come with unrestricted~~ of hES cell research that falls outside federal funding of this research, these guidelines will continue to offer reassurance to the public and to Congress that the scientific community is attentive to ethical concerns and is capable of self-regulation while moving forward with this important research.

To help ensure that these guidelines are taken seriously, stakeholders in hES cell research—sponsors, funding sources, research institutions, relevant oversight committees, professional societies, and scientific journals, as well as investigators—should develop policies and practices that are consistent with the principles inherent in these guidelines. Funding agencies, professional societies, journals, and institutional review panels can provide valuable community pressure and impose appropriate sanctions to ensure compliance. For example, ESCROs and IRBs should require evidence of compliance when protocols are reviewed for renewal, funding agencies should assess compliance when reviewing applications for support, and journals should require that evidence of compliance accompanies publication of results.

As individual states and private entities move increasingly into hES cell research, it will be important to initiate a national effort to provide a formal context in which the complex moral and oversight questions associated with this work can be addressed on a continuing basis. Both the state of hES cell research and clinical practice and public policy surrounding these topics are in a state of flux and are likely to be so for several years. Therefore, the committee believes that ~~a national body~~ mechanisms should be established to assess periodically the adequacy of the policies and guidelines proposed in this document and elsewhere and to provide a forum for a continuing discussion of issues involved in hES cell research. New policies and standards may be appropriate for issues that cannot now be foreseen. The organization that sponsors this body should be politically independent and without conflicts of interest, should be respected in the lay and scientific communities, and able to call on suitable expertise to support this effort.

Appendix D

Committee Member and Staff Biographies

COCHAIRS

R. Alta Charo, JD, is the Warren P. Knowles Professor of Law and Bioethics at the University of Wisconsin–Madison, on the faculties of both the Law School and the Medical School. On August 31, 2009, she took leave to serve as a senior policy advisor in the Office of the Commissioner of the U.S. Food and Drug Administration. Professor Charo is the author of nearly 100 articles, book chapters, and government reports on such topics as voting rights, environmental law, family planning and abortion law, medical genetics law, reproductive technology policy, science policy, and medical ethics. She has been a member of the boards of the Alan Guttmacher Institute and the Foundation for Genetic Medicine, a member of the National Medical Advisory Committee of the Planned Parenthood Federation of America, and a member of the ethics advisory boards of the International Society for Stem Cell Research, the Juvenile Diabetes Research Foundation, and WiCell. In 1994, Professor Charo served on the National Institutes of Health Human Embryo Research Panel, and from 1996 to 2001, she was a member of the presidential National Bioethics Advisory Commission. She was a member of the National Academies' Board on Life Sciences from 2001 until 2007 and since 2006 has been a member of the Institute of Medicine (IOM) Board on Population Health and Public Health Practices. Professor Charo was elected to IOM in 2006.

Richard O. Hynes, PhD, is the Daniel K. Ludwig Professor for Cancer Research at the David H. Koch Institute for Integrative Cancer Research and Department of Biology at MIT and a Howard Hughes Medical Institute Investigator. He was formerly head of the Biology Department and then director of the Center for Cancer Research at the Massachusetts Institute of Technology. His research focuses on fibronectins and integrins and the molecular basis of cellular adhesion, both in normal development and in pathological situations, such as cancer, thrombosis, and inflammation. Dr. Hynes's current interests are cancer invasion and metastasis, angiogenesis, and animal models of human disease states. He is a member of the National Academy of Sciences and the Institute of Medicine and is a fellow of the Royal Society of London and the American Academy of Arts and Sciences. In 1997, he received the Gairdner International Foundation Award. In 2000, he served as president of the American Society for Cell Biology and testified before Congress about the need for federal support and oversight of embryonic stem cell research. He cochaired the 2005 National Academies *Guidelines for Human Embryonic Stem Cell Research* and is a governor of the Wellcome Trust, UK.

MEMBERS

Eli Y. Adashi, MD, MS, CPE, FACOG, is professor of medical science and the immediate past dean of medicine and biological sciences and the Frank L. Day Professor of Biology at Brown University. Harvard-educated in Health Care Management (MS, 2005), Dr. Adashi previously served as the John A. Dixon Endowed Presidential Professor and Chair of the Department of Obstetrics and Gynecology at the University of Utah Health Sciences Center. A member of the Council on Foreign Relations, the Council on Population Growth of the World Economic Forum, the Association of American Physicians, the Royal College of Obstetricians and Gynaecologists (ad Eundem), and the American Association for the Advancement of Science, Dr. Adashi is a veteran practitioner of women's health. An adviser to the World Health Organization, the World Bank, the Rockefeller Foundation and the Bill and Melinda Gates Foundation, Dr. Adashi is a recent Franklin fellow and Senior Advisor on Global Women's Health to the Secretary of State Office of Global Women's Issues headed by Ambassador-At-Large Melanne Verveer. A long-standing NIH-funded scientist and a Research Career Development Awardee, Dr. Adashi is a former Donna Shalala appointee to the National Advisory Council of the Eunice Kennedy Shriver National Institute of Child

Health and Human Development (NICHD). In addition, Dr. Adashi served the NIH as a member of the Reproductive Sciences 5-Year Planning Forum for NICHD, as a member of the selection committee of the Reproductive Scientist Development Program and as a member of the Reproductive Endocrinology Study Section. A former president of the Society for Reproductive Endocrinologists, the Society for Gynecologic Investigation, and the American Gynecological and Obstetrical Society, Dr. Adashi is the author or co-author of over 250 peer-reviewed publications, over 120 book chapters/reviews, and 13 books focusing on ovarian biology, ovarian cancer and women's reproductive health, freedom and rights. Elected to the Institute of Medicine in 1999, Adashi served on consensus committees on Women's Health Research, Antiprogestins: Assessing the Science and Understanding Premature Birth and Assuring Health Outcomes. Dr. Adashi has also served the IOM as a reviewer of *New Frontiers in Contraceptive Research, A Comprehensive Review of the DHHS Office of Family Planning Title X Program* and *Policy Issues in the Development of Personalized Medicine in Oncology*. Dr. Adashi is presently serving on the Board of Directors of Physicians for Human Rights and Population Connection as well as on the Board of Governors of Tel Aviv University.

A native of Israel, Dr. Adashi received his medical degree in 1973 from the Sackler School of Medicine of Tel Aviv University. After serving a straight medical internship in the same, Dr. Adashi (a naturalized U.S. citizen) completed residency training in obstetrics and gynecology at the New England Medical Center of Tufts University (1974-77). Fellowship training in the subspecialty of reproductive endocrinology and postdoctoral training in reproductive biology followed suit at Johns Hopkins University and at the University of California at San Diego, respectively (1977-81).

Brigid L.M. Hogan, PhD, is the George Barth Geller Professor and chair of the Department of Cell Biology, Duke University Medical Center. Before joining Duke, Dr. Hogan was an investigator of the Howard Hughes Medical Institute and Hortense B. Ingram Professor in the Department of Cell Biology at Vanderbilt University Medical Center. Dr. Hogan earned her PhD in biochemistry at the University of Cambridge. She was then a postdoctoral fellow in the Department of Biology at the Massachusetts Institute of Technology. Before moving to the United States in 1988, Dr. Hogan was head of the Molecular Embryology Laboratory at the National Institute for Medical Research in London. Her research focuses on the genetic control of embryonic development and morphogenesis, using the mouse as a model system. Her laboratory developed methods for deriving mouse pluripotential embryonic germ cell lines. She was co-chair for science of the 1994 National Institutes of Health Human Embryo Research Panel and a member of the 2001-2002 National Academies Panel on Scientific and Medical Aspects of Human Cloning. Within the last few years, Dr. Hogan has been elected to the Royal Society of London, the American Academy of Arts and Sciences, the Institute of Medicine, and the National Academy of Sciences.

Marcia Imbrescia is the owner of Peartree Design, a landscape design firm, and was previously the media director for Drumbeater, a high-technology advertising agency. She holds BA degrees in marketing and journalism and a graduate certificate in landscape design. Ms. Imbrescia has a passion for health advocacy and helping people with illness and disability. She is a past member of the Board of Trustees of the Arthritis Foundation (AF) (2003-2007), for which she has participated as a volunteer at the chapter and national levels. She served as a member (1996-1998 and 2001) and chairperson (2002-2003) of AF's American Juvenile Arthritis Organization. In 1992, she received the Volunteer of the Year Award from the Massachusetts Chapter of AF. Her volunteer efforts include program development, conference planning, public speaking, fundraising, and advocacy. Currently, Ms. Imbrescia is an active volunteer with New England Disabled Sports. She served on the National Academies Committee on Guidelines for Human Embryonic Stem Cell Research in 2004-2005.

Terry Magnuson, PhD, is Sarah Graham Kenan Professor and chair of the Department of Genetics at the University of North Carolina. He also directs the Carolina Center for Genome Sciences and is the program director of cancer genetics at the Lineberger Comprehensive Cancer Center. Dr. Magnuson's research interests include mammalian genetics, genomics, and development. His laboratory has developed a high-throughput system to study the effects of mutations on mouse development with mouse embryonic stem cells. He is particularly interested in the role of chromatin remodeling complexes in such processes as autosomal imprinting, X-inactivation, and anterior-posterior patterning of axial structures in mammals. He is an elected member of the American Academy of Arts and Sciences and was a member of the Board of Directors of the Genetics Society of America and of the Society for Developmental Biology.

Linda B. Miller, OTR, MS in hospital administration, is president of the Washington, DC–based Volunteer Trustees Foundation, a consortium of not-for-profit hospital governing boards. She has extensive experience in trustee education, advocacy, and the legal, ethical, and policy issues facing voluntary health care institutions. Recently, she has worked closely with the states' attorneys general in developing guidelines for protecting the community interest in the sale and conversion of nonprofit hospitals and in designing models for practice and legal oversight. She was elected to membership in the Institute of Medicine (IOM) in 1997.

Ms. Miller has been a frequent speaker on health-policy issues and has been published extensively in both the medical and popular press, including the *New England Journal of Medicine*, *Health Affairs*, *USA Today*, the *Washington Post,* and the *New York Times*. She served as a special assistant to the secretary of health, education, and welfare (now the Department of Health and Human Services) and on numerous health-related policy councils and advisory committees, including the National Institutes of Health's Consensus Panel on Liver Transplantation and, most recently, IOM's Committee on Spinal Cord Injury. Ms. Miller serves on the Advisory Board of the University of Louisville–based Institute for Cellular Therapeutics, headed by Suzanne Ildstad, which does research in adult bone marrow transplantation, and has been a member of several academic and health-care institutions' boards of governors, including those of Blythedale Children's Hospital in New York, Capital Hospice in the national capital region, and Cornell University's Alumni Council.

Jonathan D. Moreno, PhD, is the David and Lyn Silfen University Professor of Ethics and professor of medical ethics and of the history and sociology of science at the University of Pennsylvania. He holds a courtesy appointment as professor of philosophy. He is also a senior fellow at the Center for American Progress in Washington, D.C., where edits the magazine *Science Progress* (www.scienceprogress.org). He was a member of President Barack Obama's transition team for the Department of Health and Human Services. Moreno is an elected member of the Institute of Medicine/National Academy of Sciences. In 2008 he was designated a National Associate of the National Research Council. He has served as a senior staff member for two presidential advisory commissions, and has given invited testimony for both houses of congress. He was an Andrew W. Mellon post doctoral fellow, holds an honorary doctorate from Hofstra University, and is a recipient of the Benjamin Rush Medal from the College of William and Mary Law School. Moreno has served as adviser to the Howard Hughes Medical Institute and the Bill and Melinda Gates Foundation, among many other organizations. Moreno is also a faculty affiliate of the Kennedy Institute of Ethics at Georgetown University and a fellow of the Hastings Center and the New York Academy of Medicine. He is a past president of the American Society for Bioethics and Humanities. His books include *Progress in Bioethics* (2010); *Science Next: Innovation for the Common Good* (2009); *Mind Wars: Brain Research and National Defense* (2006); *Undue Risk: Secret State Experiments on Humans* (1999); *Ethical Guidelines for Innovative Surgery (2006); Is There an Ethicist in the House?* (2005); *In the Wake of Terror: Medicine and Morality in a Time of Crisis* (2003); *Ethical and Regulatory Aspects of Clinical Research* (2003); *Deciding Together: Bioethics and Moral Consensus* (1995); *Ethics in Clinical Practice* (2000); and *Arguing Euthanasia* (1995). Moreno has published more than 300 papers, reviews and book chapters, and is a member of several editorial boards.

Pilar N. Ossorio, PhD, JD, is associate professor of law and bioethics at the University of Wisconsin–Madison and program faculty in the Graduate Program in Population Health at the university. Before taking her position there, she was director of the Genetics Section of the Institute for Ethics at the American Medical Association and taught as an adjunct faculty member at the University of Chicago Law School. For the 2006 calendar year, Professor Ossorio was a visiting professor of law at the University of California, Berkeley Boalt Hall School of Law.

Dr. Ossorio received her PhD in microbiology and immunology in 1990 from Stanford University. She went on to complete a postdoctoral fellowship in cell biology at Yale University School of Medicine. Throughout the early 1990s, Dr. Ossorio worked as a consultant for the federal program on the Ethical, Legal, and Social Implications (ELSI) of the Human Genome Project; in 1994, she took a full-time position with the Department of Energy's ELSI program. In 1993, she served on the Ethics Working Group for President Clinton's Health Care Reform Task Force. Dr. Ossorio received her JD from the Boalt Hall School of Law in 1997. While there, she was elected to the legal honor society Order of the Coif and received several awards for outstanding legal scholarship.

Dr. Ossorio is a fellow of the American Association for the Advancement of Science (AAAS), on the Editorial Board of the *American Journal of Bioethics*, an adviser to the National Human Genome Research Institute on ethical issues in large-scale sequencing, and a member of the University of Wisconsin's institutional review board for health-sciences research. She is a past member of AAAS's Committee on Scientific Freedom and Responsibility, a past member of the National Cancer Policy Board in the Institute of Medicine, and a past member or chair of several working groups on genetics and ethics. She has published scholarly articles in bioethics, law, and molecular biology.

E. Albert Reece, MD, PhD, is dean of the University of Maryland School of Medicine and vice president for medical affairs at the University of Maryland, Baltimore. Previously, he was vice chancellor and dean of the University of Arkansas College of Medicine. Dr. Reece received his undergraduate degree from Long Island University, his MD (Magna Cum Laude) from New York University, his PhD in biochemistry from the University of the West Indies, and his MBA from the Fox School of Business and Management of Temple University. He completed a residency in obstetrics and gynecology at Columbia University–Presbyterian Hospital and a fellowship in maternal-fetal medicine at Yale University School of Medicine. He served on the faculty at Yale for 10 years and was the chairman of the Department of Obstetrics, Gynecology and Reproductive Sciences at Temple University. Dr. Reece has published over 400 journal articles, book chapters, and abstracts and nine textbooks, including *Diabetes in Pregnancy, Medicine of the Fetus & Mother,* and *Fundamentals of Obstetric & Gynecologic Ultrasound.* He is an editor for the *Journal of Maternal-Fetal Medicine* and a reviewer for several other scientific journals. His research focuses on diabetes in pregnancy, birth defects, and prenatal diagnosis. Dr. Reece is a member of the Institute of Medicine.

Joshua R. Sanes, PhD, is professor of molecular and cellular biology and the Paul J. Finnegan Family Director of the Center for Brain Science at Harvard University. He was previously Alumni Endowed Professor of Neurobiology at the Washington University School of Medicine. Dr. Sanes earned a BA in biochemistry and psychology at Yale and a PhD in Neurobiology at Harvard. He studies the formation of the synapses that interconnect nerve cells, including pioneering work on the signals exchanged between nerve cells and their target muscles as new connections are made. He is also using the vertebrate visual system to examine how nerve cells develop and migrate to the right location in the body. He has been elected a fellow of the American Association for the Advancement of Science and a member of the National Academy of Sciences and the American Academy of Arts and Sciences.

Harold T. Shapiro, PhD, is president emeritus of both Princeton University and the University of Michigan and is currently professor of economics and public affairs at Princeton University. His research interests include bioethics, the social role of higher education, hospital and medical- center administration, university administration, econometrics, statistics, and economics. Dr. Shapiro chaired the Board of Trustees of the Alfred P. Sloan Foundation, was presiding director for the Dow Chemical Company, and is a member of numerous boards, including the Robert Wood Johnson Medical School, HCA, the Merck Vaccine Advisory Board, the Knight Foundation Commission on Intercollegiate Athletics, the U.S. Olympic Committee, and the Stem Cell Institute of New Jersey. He is a former chair of the Association of American Universities and the National Bioethics Advisory Committee and vice chair of the President's Council of Advisors on Science and Technology. He has also served on the Board of Directors of the National Bureau of Economic Research, Inc. and the Board of Trustees of the Universities Research Association, Inc. He has chaired and served on numerous National Academies committees, including the Committee on the Organizational Structure of the National Institutes of Health and the Committee on Particle Physics. Dr. Shapiro was named the 2006 American Association for the Advancement of Science William D. Carey Lecturer for his leadership in science policy. He earned a PhD in economics from Princeton University and holds 14 honorary doctorates.

John E. Wagner, Jr., MD, is a professor of pediatrics at the University of Minnesota Medical School. He is the first recipient of the Children's Cancer Research Fund/Hageboeck Family Chair in Pediatric Oncology and also holds the University of Minnesota McKnight Presidential Chair in Cancer Research. He is the director of the Division of Pediatric Hematology/Oncology and Bone Marrow Transplantation and scientific director of clinical research of the Stem Cell Institute. Dr. Wagner is a member of numerous societies, including the American Society of Hematology, the International Society of Experimental Hematology, and the American Society of Blood and Marrow Transplantation. He is a member of several honorary societies, including Alpha Omega Alpha (1980), the American Society of Clinical Investigation (2000), and the Association of American Physicians (2006). Dr. Wagner holds a patent on the isolation of the pluripotential quiescent stem cell population. Dr. Wagner holds a BA in biological sciences and a BA in psychology from the University of Delaware and an MD from Jefferson Medical College. Dr. Wagner's research has focused on the development of novel cellular therapies for tissue repair and suppression of the immune response using subpopulations of neonatal umbilical cord blood and adult bone marrow and peripheral blood. His projects are funded by the National Institutes of Health and industry. In addition, Dr. Wagner pioneered the use of embryo selection to "create" a perfectly tissue-matched stem cell donor for the treatment of genetic disease. Dr. Wagner has written more than 250 articles and book chapters in the field of hematopoietic stem cell transplantation. He previously served as a member of the Scientific Board of Directors of the National Marrow Donor Program and on the Institute of Medicine's Committee on Establishing a National Cord Blood Stem Cell Banking Program. He is currently a member of the Scientific and Medical Accountability Standards Working Group of the California Institute of Regenerative Medicine.

STAFF

Adam P. Fagen, PhD, is a senior program officer with the Board on Life Sciences of the National Research Council. He came to the National Academies from Harvard University, where he most recently served as preceptor on molecular and cellular biology. He earned his PhD in molecular biology and education from Harvard, working on issues related to undergraduate science courses; his research focused on mechanisms for assessing and enhancing introductory science courses in biology and physics to encourage student learning and conceptual understanding, including studies of active learning, classroom demonstrations, and student understanding of genetics vocabulary. Dr. Fagen also received an AM in molecular and cellular biology from Harvard, based on laboratory research in molecular evolutionary genetics, and a BA from Swarthmore College with a double-major in biology and mathematics. He served as co-director of the 2000 National Doctoral Program Survey, an on-line assessment of doctoral programs organized by the National Association of Graduate-Professional Students, supported by the Alfred P. Sloan Foundation, and completed by over 32,000 students.

At the National Academies, Dr. Fagen has served as study director for *Bridges to Independence: Fostering the Independence of New Investigators in Biomedical Research* (2005), *Treating Infectious Diseases in a Microbial World: Report of Two Workshops on Novel Antimicrobial Therapeutics* (2006), *2007* and *2008 Amendments to the National Academies' Guidelines for Human Embryonic Stem Cell Research* (2007, 2008), *Understanding Interventions that Encourage Minorities to Pursue Research Careers: Summary of a Workshop* (2007), *Inspired by Biology: From Molecules to Materials to Machines* (2008), *Transforming Agricultural Education for a Changing World* (2009), *Responsible Research with Biological Select Agents and Toxins* (2009), and *Research at the Intersection of the Physical and Life Sciences* (2010). He is currently study director or responsible staff officer for several ongoing projects including the National Academies Summer

Institute on Undergraduate Education in Biology, the National Academies Human Embryonic Stem Cell Research Advisory Committee, and the Special Immunizations Program for Laboratory Personnel Engaged in Research on Countermeasures for Select Agents.

Bruce M. Altevogt, PhD, is a senior program officer in the Board on Health Sciences Policy at the Institute of Medicine (IOM). His primary interests focus on policy issues related to basic research and preparedness for catastrophic events. He received his doctoral thesis from Harvard University's Program in Neuroscience. Following over 10 years of research, Dr. Altevogt joined The National Academies as a science and technology policy fellow with the Christine Mirzayan Science & Technology Policy Graduate Fellowship Program. Since joining the Board on Health Sciences Policy, he has been a program officer on multiple IOM studies including, *Sleep Disorders and Sleep Deprivation: An Unmet Public Health Problem, The National Academies' Guidelines for Human Embryonic Stem Cell Research: 2007 Amendments* and *2008 Amendments, and Research Priorities in Emergency Preparedness and Response for Public Health Systems.* He is currently serving as the director of the Forum on Medical and Public Health Preparedness for Catastrophic Events, the Neuroscience and Nervous System Disorders Forum, and as a co-study director on the National Academies Human Embryonic Stem Cells Research Advisory Committee. He received his BA from the University of Virginia in Charlottesville, where he majored in biology and minored in South Asian studies.

Frances E. Sharples, PhD, has served as director of the National Research Council's Board on Life Sciences since October 2000. Immediately prior to this position, she was a senior policy analyst for the Environment Division of the White House Office of Science and Technology Policy (OSTP) for four years. Dr. Sharples came to OSTP from the Oak Ridge National Laboratory, where she served in various positions in the Environmental Sciences Division between 1978 and 1996, most recently as a Research and Development Section Head. Dr. Sharples received her BA in biology from Barnard College and her MA and PhD in zoology from the University of California, Davis. She served as an American Association for the Advancement of Science (AAAS) Environmental Science and Engineering Fellow at the Environmental Protection Agency during the summer of 1981, and served as a AAAS Congressional Science and Engineering Fellow in the office of Senator Al Gore in 1984-85. She was a member of the National Institutes of Health's

Recombinant DNA Advisory Committee in the mid-1980s, and was elected a Fellow of the AAAS in 1992.

Andrew M. Pope, PhD, is director of the Board on Health Sciences Policy in the Institute of Medicine (IOM). He has a PhD in physiology and biochemistry from the University of Maryland and has been a member of the National Academies staff since 1982 and of the IOM staff since 1989. His primary interests are science policy, biomedical ethics, and environmental and occupational influences on human health. During his tenure at the National Academies, Dr. Pope has directed numerous studies on topics that range from injury control, disability prevention, and biologic markers to the protection of human subjects of research, National Institutes of Health priority-setting processes, organ procurement and transplantation policy, and the role of science and technology in countering terrorism. Dr. Pope is the recipient of IOM's Cecil Award and the National Academy of Sciences President's Special Achievement Award.

Amanda P. Cline, is a senior program assistant with the Board on Life Sciences at the National Academies. She earned a BS in environmental studies from Bucknell University in 2006.